MIDNIGHT LIGHTS PUBLISHING HOUSE

PRESENTS:

WORLD'S BEST MOTHER

ACTIVE MOMS

AUTHOR OF THE BOOK:

RACHEL GUARDIAN

TABLE OF CONTENTS

Introduction to Exercise During Pregnancy...

Benefits of Staying Active During Pregnancy....................................

Safe Exercises During Pregnancy......................................1

Precautions and Guidelines for Exercising Safely.............................19

Nutrition and Hydration During Exercise...............................24

Managing Common Pregnancy Discomforts Through Exercise........30

Exercise Modifications for Each Trimester..............................36

Postpartum Exercise and Recovery....................................41

Real-life Stories and Testimonials.....................................47

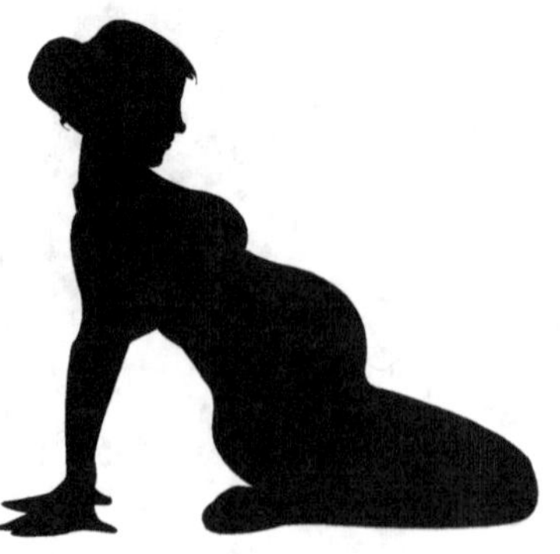

Introduction to Exercise During Pregnancy

Introduction to Exercise During Pregnancy

Pregnancy is a transformative journey marked by physical, emotional, and psychological changes. Amidst these changes, the importance of maintaining an active lifestyle cannot be overstated. In this chapter, we explore the significance of exercise during pregnancy and the multitude of benefits it offers for both the mother and baby.

Why Exercise Matters

During pregnancy, a woman's body undergoes profound changes to accommodate the growing fetus. These changes include hormonal fluctuations, weight gain, postural adjustments, and increased strain on various bodily systems. While it's natural to experience discomfort and fatigue during this time, staying physically active can help alleviate many of these symptoms.

Contrary to common misconceptions, exercise during pregnancy is not only safe but also highly beneficial when done in moderation and under appropriate guidance. Research has shown that regular exercise can improve cardiovascular health, enhance muscle tone and strength, and promote overall well-being. Additionally, staying active can help manage common discomforts such as back pain, swelling, and constipation, thereby enhancing the quality of life for pregnant individuals.

Physical Benefits

The physical benefits of exercise during pregnancy are manifold. Engaging in regular physical activity helps maintain cardiovascular fitness, which is crucial for supporting the increased demands placed on the heart and circulatory system during pregnancy. Furthermore, exercises that target the core and pelvic floor muscles can help improve stability, balance, and posture, reducing the risk of musculoskeletal issues such as lower back pain and pelvic girdle pain.

Exercise also plays a vital role in managing weight gain during pregnancy. By promoting healthy weight management, physical activity can help reduce the risk of gestational diabetes and hypertensive disorders, both of which are associated with maternal obesity and excessive weight gain during pregnancy.

Psychological Benefits

In addition to the physical benefits, exercise during pregnancy offers significant psychological advantages. Pregnancy is often accompanied by heightened emotions, anxiety, and stress, which can take a toll on mental well-being. Engaging in regular exercise provides an outlet for stress relief, promotes relaxation, and boosts mood-enhancing endorphins, helping pregnant individuals cope with the emotional challenges of pregnancy.

Moreover, exercise fosters a sense of empowerment and confidence, enabling pregnant individuals to connect with their bodies and embrace the changes they are experiencing. This newfound sense of control and self-assurance can have a profound impact on self-esteem and body image during pregnancy and beyond.

Benefits for the Baby

While much of the focus is understandably on the mother's health during pregnancy, it's important to recognize that maternal well-being directly influences fetal development and long-term health outcomes for the baby. Research suggests that maternal exercise can positively impact fetal development by improving placental function, optimizing nutrient delivery, and enhancing oxygenation of the developing fetus.

Furthermore, maternal exercise has been associated with improved neonatal outcomes, including reduced rates of preterm birth and low birth weight. By promoting a healthy intrauterine environment, exercise during pregnancy sets the stage for optimal growth and development, laying the foundation for a healthy start to life.

Conclusion

In conclusion, exercise during pregnancy is not only safe but also highly beneficial for both the mother and baby. By embracing physical activity as part of their prenatal care regimen, pregnant individuals can experience improved physical fitness, enhanced emotional well-being, and better pregnancy outcomes. In the chapters that follow, we will delve into specific exercises, safety precautions, and practical tips for incorporating exercise into pregnancy, empowering readers to embark on a journey of health and vitality during this transformative time.

Benefits of Staying Active During Pregnancy

Staying active during pregnancy offers a multitude of benefits for both the mother and baby. In this chapter, we'll explore the physical and psychological advantages for the mother, as well as the benefits for the baby's development.

Physical Benefits for the Mother

- Improved Cardiovascular Health: Regular physical activity during pregnancy helps maintain cardiovascular fitness, supporting the increased demands placed on the heart and circulatory system. Engaging in aerobic exercise can improve circulation, lower blood pressure, and reduce the risk of cardiovascular complications.

- Enhanced Muscular Strength and Endurance: Strength training exercises help strengthen the muscles of the body, including the core, back, and pelvic floor muscles. Strong muscles provide better support for the growing uterus and help alleviate common discomforts such as back pain and pelvic instability.
- Better Weight Management: Exercise can help manage weight gain during pregnancy by promoting healthy weight maintenance and preventing excessive weight gain. This reduces the risk of gestational diabetes, preeclampsia, and other complications associated with maternal obesity.

- Increased Energy Levels: Staying active boosts energy levels and reduces fatigue, allowing pregnant women to better cope with the physical demands of pregnancy and daily activities. Regular exercise also improves sleep quality, leading to better overall well-being.

Psychological Benefits for the Mother

- Reduced Stress and Anxiety: Exercise triggers the release of endorphins, the body's natural mood elevators, which help reduce stress and anxiety levels. Physical activity also provides a distraction from worries and promotes a sense of relaxation and well-being.
- Improved Mood and Emotional Well-being: Engaging in regular exercise enhances mood, increases self-esteem, and promotes a positive outlook on pregnancy and motherhood. Physical activity

stimulates the production of neurotransmitters such as serotonin and dopamine, which contribute to feelings of happiness and contentment.

- Enhanced Body Image and Self-confidence: Pregnancy brings about changes in the body that can affect self-esteem and body image. By staying active, women can maintain a sense of control over their bodies, feel more confident in their physical abilities, and embrace the changes associated with pregnancy.
- Social Support and Connection: Participating in prenatal exercise classes or group activities provides an opportunity to connect with other pregnant women and share experiences. Building a support network of like-minded individuals can provide encouragement, motivation, and camaraderie throughout the pregnancy journey.

Benefits for the Baby

- Improved Placental Function:
  Maternal exercise has been shown
  to enhance placental function,
  leading to better nutrient delivery
  and oxygenation of the developing
  fetus. A healthy placenta supports
  optimal fetal growth and
  development throughout
  pregnancy.
- Enhanced Fetal
  Neurodevelopment: Research
  suggests that maternal exercise
  may have a positive impact on fetal
  neurodevelopment, including
  cognitive and motor skills. Regular
  physical activity during pregnancy
  may contribute to improved brain
  development and cognitive
  functioning in the offspring.
- Reduced Risk of Pregnancy
  Complications: Maternal exercise
  has been associated with a
  reduced risk of pregnancy
  complications such as gestational

diabetes, preeclampsia, and preterm birth. By promoting maternal health and well-being, exercise creates a more favorable intrauterine environment for the baby.

- Long-Term Health Benefits: The benefits of maternal exercise extend beyond pregnancy and childbirth, influencing the long-term health outcomes of the offspring. Children born to physically active mothers may have a lower risk of obesity, cardiovascular disease, and metabolic disorders later in life.

Safe Exercises During Pregnancy

During pregnancy, maintaining an active lifestyle is important for promoting overall health and well-being. However, it's essential to choose exercises that are safe and appropriate for this unique stage of life. In this chapter, we'll explore a variety of safe exercises tailored specifically for pregnant individuals, including low-impact cardio, strength training with modifications, and flexibility and stretching exercises.

Low-Impact Cardio Exercises

Cardiovascular exercise is an excellent way to improve endurance, boost mood, and maintain cardiovascular health during pregnancy. Low-impact cardio exercises are particularly well-suited for pregnant individuals as they minimize stress on the joints while providing effective cardiovascular benefits. Here are some safe and enjoyable low-impact cardio exercises for pregnant women:

- Walking: Brisk walking is one of the simplest and most accessible forms of exercise during pregnancy. Aim to walk for at least 30 minutes most days of the week, gradually increasing the duration and intensity as tolerated.

- Swimming: Swimming is a low-impact, full-body workout that offers cardiovascular benefits without putting strain on the joints. Water provides buoyancy and support, making it an ideal exercise for pregnant individuals, especially those experiencing discomfort or swelling.
- Stationary Cycling: Riding a stationary bike is a safe and effective way to get your heart rate up during pregnancy. Adjust the resistance and pace to a comfortable level, and avoid standing while cycling to prevent strain on the pelvis and lower back.
- Prenatal Aerobics Classes: Many fitness centers offer prenatal aerobics classes specifically designed for pregnant women.

These classes typically include low-impact cardio exercises, as well as strength training and flexibility exercises tailored to the needs of expectant mothers.

Remember to listen to your body and modify exercises as needed. Stay hydrated, wear supportive footwear, and avoid overheating. If you experience any discomfort, dizziness, or shortness of breath, stop exercising and consult with your healthcare provider.

Strength Training Exercises with Modifications

Maintaining muscle strength and tone is important during pregnancy, as it can help support the changing body and prepare for labor and delivery. However, traditional strength training exercises may need to be modified to accommodate the physical changes of pregnancy. Here are some safe strength training exercises with modifications for pregnant individuals:

- Squats: Squats are a great way to strengthen the lower body, including the quadriceps, hamstrings, and glutes. To perform a squat safely during pregnancy, keep your feet hip-width apart, lower your body as if sitting back into a chair, and avoid squatting too low to prevent strain on the pelvic floor.
- Modified Push-Ups: Push-ups are an effective upper body exercise that can be modified to accommodate a growing belly. Perform push-ups against a wall or using an elevated surface, such as a countertop or sturdy chair, to reduce strain on the core and abdominal muscles.
- Pelvic Floor Exercises: Strengthening the pelvic floor muscles is particularly important during pregnancy and can help

prevent urinary incontinence and support the growing uterus. Kegel exercises, which involve contracting and relaxing the pelvic floor muscles, can be performed anywhere, anytime throughout the day.

- Resistance Band Exercises: Resistance bands are versatile tools that can be used to perform a variety of strength training exercises during pregnancy. Choose a light to moderate resistance band and incorporate exercises such as bicep curls, shoulder presses, and rows into your routine.

Focus on maintaining proper form, breathing rhythmically, and avoiding exercises that involve lying flat on your back after the first trimester. If you're unsure about which exercises are safe for you, consult with a certified prenatal fitness instructor or physical therapist for personalized guidance.

Flexibility and Stretching Exercises

Flexibility and stretching exercises are essential for maintaining range of motion, improving posture, and reducing muscle tension during pregnancy. Gentle stretching can also help alleviate common discomforts such as back pain and tightness. Here are some safe flexibility and stretching exercises for pregnant individuals:

- Cat-Cow Stretch: Start on your hands and knees, with your wrists aligned under your shoulders and your knees under your hips. Inhale as you arch your back and lift your head and tailbone toward the ceiling (cat pose), then exhale as you round your back and tuck your chin to your chest (cow pose). Repeat for several breaths, moving fluidly between the two poses.
- Seated Forward Bend: Sit on the floor with your legs extended in front of you and your feet flexed.

Inhale as you lengthen your spine, then exhale as you hinge forward from your hips, reaching toward your toes. Hold the stretch for 15-30 seconds, breathing deeply into the stretch, then slowly release.

- Prenatal Yoga: Prenatal yoga classes often include a variety of stretching exercises and gentle yoga poses tailored specifically for pregnant women. These poses help improve flexibility, strengthen the body, and promote relaxation and stress relief.

- Hip Opener Stretches: Pregnancy can cause tightness and tension in the hips and pelvis. Incorporate hip opener stretches such as pigeon pose, seated figure-four stretch, and butterfly stretch into your routine to release tension and improve mobility in the hips.

Avoid overstretching or bouncing during stretches, and listen to your body's cues to avoid discomfort or pain. As your pregnancy progresses, you may need to modify your stretching routine to accommodate your changing body and avoid positions that feel uncomfortable or unstable.

Precautions and Guidelines for Exercising Safely

Exercising during pregnancy offers numerous benefits, but it's essential to prioritize safety and well-being. In this chapter, we'll discuss precautions and guidelines to help pregnant individuals exercise safely, including consulting with a healthcare provider, monitoring intensity and heart rate, and recognizing signs to stop exercising and seek medical attention.

Consulting with a Healthcare Provider

Before starting or continuing an exercise routine during pregnancy, it's important to consult with a healthcare provider, such as an obstetrician or midwife. Your healthcare provider can assess your individual health status, pregnancy risk factors, and any medical conditions that may impact your ability to exercise safely.

During the consultation, be sure to discuss:

- Your current exercise routine and activity level
- Any medical conditions or pregnancy complications
- Previous pregnancies or childbirth experiences
- Any concerns or questions you may have about exercising during pregnancy

Your healthcare provider can provide personalized guidance and recommendations based on your individual health needs and pregnancy status. They may also refer you to a certified prenatal fitness instructor or physical therapist for additional support and guidance.

Monitoring Intensity and Heart Rate

During pregnancy, it's important to monitor exercise intensity and heart rate to ensure that you're exercising safely and effectively. While the American College of Obstetricians and Gynecologists (ACOG) recommends moderate-intensity exercise for most pregnant women, individual tolerance may vary.

To monitor exercise intensity:

- Use the "talk test" to gauge your exertion level. If you can carry on a conversation while exercising without feeling breathless, you're likely exercising at a moderate intensity.
- Pay attention to your perceived exertion level on a scale of 1 to 10,

with 1 being very light activity and
10 being maximal exertion. Aim to
keep your exertion level between 3
and 5 during exercise.
- Avoid overexertion or pushing
yourself to the point of exhaustion.
Pregnancy is not the time to set
personal records or engage in
high-intensity workouts.

Additionally, monitor your heart rate
during exercise and aim to keep it within
a safe range. The ACOG recommends that
pregnant women avoid exercising at heart
rates above 140 beats per minute,
although individual recommendations
may vary based on fitness level and
pregnancy status.

**Signs to Stop Exercising and Seek
Medical Attention**

While exercise is generally safe during
pregnancy, there are certain signs and
symptoms that indicate it's time to stop

exercising and seek medical attention.
These may include:

- Vaginal bleeding or spotting
- Severe abdominal pain or cramping
- Persistent dizziness or lightheadedness
- Shortness of breath that doesn't resolve with rest
- Chest pain or palpitations
- Decreased fetal movement or unusual fetal activity

If you experience any of these symptoms during exercise, stop exercising immediately and consult with your healthcare provider. It's important to listen to your body and prioritize safety throughout your pregnancy journey.

Nutrition and Hydration During Exercise

Proper nutrition and hydration are essential components of a healthy pregnancy, particularly when engaging in exercise. In this chapter, we'll explore the importance of maintaining adequate nutrition and hydration during pregnancy, along with guidelines for optimizing pre- and post-workout nutrition.

Importance of Proper Nutrition During Pregnancy

Nutrition plays a crucial role in supporting maternal health and fetal development during pregnancy. Expectant mothers require additional nutrients to meet the needs of both themselves and their growing baby.

Proper nutrition during pregnancy can help:

- Support Fetal Growth and Development: Nutrients such as folate, iron, calcium, and protein are essential for fetal growth and development. Adequate intake of these nutrients during pregnancy is crucial for preventing birth defects, promoting healthy birth weight, and ensuring optimal development of the baby's organs and tissues.
- Maintain Maternal Health: Pregnancy places increased demands on the mother's body, requiring additional nutrients to support maternal health and well-being. Proper nutrition during pregnancy can help prevent complications such as gestational diabetes, preeclampsia, and maternal anemia, and promote overall health and vitality for the mother.

- Support Energy Levels and
  Physical Activity: Engaging in
  regular exercise during pregnancy
  requires adequate energy intake to
  fuel physical activity and support
  maternal metabolism. Proper
  nutrition provides the energy and
  nutrients needed to sustain
  exercise performance, enhance
  recovery, and maintain overall
  fitness during pregnancy.

Hydration Guidelines for Pregnant Women

Staying hydrated is essential for supporting maternal health and well-being during pregnancy, particularly when exercising. Dehydration can increase the risk of overheating, heat exhaustion, and other complications during pregnancy. Here are some hydration guidelines for pregnant women:

- Drink Plenty of Fluids: Aim to drink at least 8-10 cups (64-80 ounces) of fluids per day, or more if you're exercising or in hot weather. Water is the best choice for staying hydrated, but you can also include other hydrating beverages such as herbal tea, coconut water, and diluted fruit juice.
- Monitor Urine Color: Pay attention to the color of your urine as a simple indicator of hydration status. Pale yellow urine indicates adequate hydration, while dark yellow urine may signal dehydration and the need to drink more fluids.
- Stay Hydrated Before, During, and After Exercise: Drink water before, during, and after exercise to maintain hydration levels and replace fluids lost through sweat. Sip water regularly throughout your workout, and hydrate adequately during rest periods.

- Consider Electrolyte Intake: If you're engaging in prolonged or intense exercise, consider replenishing electrolytes lost through sweat by consuming electrolyte-rich foods or beverages, such as sports drinks or electrolyte-enhanced water.

Pre- and Post-Workout Nutrition Tips

Proper nutrition before and after exercise can help optimize performance, enhance recovery, and support overall health during pregnancy. Here are some pre- and post-workout nutrition tips for pregnant women:

- Pre-Workout Nutrition: Eat a small, balanced meal or snack containing carbohydrates and protein 1-2 hours before exercise to provide energy and fuel your workout. Examples include a banana with nut butter, yogurt

with fruit, or a small turkey
sandwich on whole grain bread.

- Post-Workout Nutrition: Refuel
  your body with a combination of
  carbohydrates and protein within
  30-60 minutes after exercise to
  support muscle recovery and
  replenish energy stores. Examples
  include a protein smoothie, Greek
  yogurt with granola, or a turkey
  and vegetable wrap.
- Listen to Your Body: Pay attention
  to hunger cues and cravings, and
  eat when you're hungry to
  replenish energy stores and
  support recovery. Choose nutrient-
  dense foods that provide a balance
  of carbohydrates, protein, healthy
  fats, vitamins, and minerals to
  meet your body's needs.

Conclusion

In conclusion, proper nutrition and
hydration are essential components of a
healthy pregnancy, particularly when

engaging in exercise. By prioritizing adequate nutrition and hydration, pregnant women can support maternal health, fetal development, and exercise performance throughout pregnancy. For more detailed information on nutrition during pregnancy, including meal planning, nutrient requirements, and healthy eating tips, refer to another book in this series called "Eat for Two."

Managing Common Pregnancy Discomforts Through Exercise

Pregnancy often brings about a range of physical discomforts, including back pain, pelvic floor issues, poor posture, and swelling. Fortunately, exercise can be an effective tool for managing these common discomforts and promoting overall comfort and well-being during pregnancy. In this chapter, we'll explore exercises specifically targeted to alleviate back pain, strengthen the pelvic floor, improve posture, and reduce swelling.

Back Pain Relief Exercises

Back pain is a common complaint among pregnant women, particularly in the later stages of pregnancy as the belly grows and the center of gravity shifts. Fortunately, gentle exercises can help alleviate back pain and improve spinal alignment. Here are some exercises to relieve back pain during pregnancy:

- Cat-Cow Stretch: Begin on your hands and knees, with your wrists aligned under your shoulders and your knees under your hips. Inhale as you arch your back and lift your head and tailbone toward the ceiling (cow pose), then exhale as you round your back and tuck your chin to your chest (cat pose). Repeat for several breaths, moving fluidly between the two poses.

- Pelvic Tilts: Lie on your back with your knees bent and your feet flat on the floor hip-width apart. Engage your abdominal muscles and tilt your pelvis slightly upward, pressing your lower back into the floor. Hold for a few seconds, then release. Repeat several times to gently stretch and strengthen the muscles of the lower back and pelvis.

- Supported Child's Pose: Begin on your hands and knees, then sit back on your heels with your knees wide apart and your forehead resting on the floor. Extend your arms forward or rest them by your sides. Place a cushion or bolster under your forehead for support. Hold the pose for several breaths, focusing on deep, diaphragmatic breathing to relax the muscles of the back and pelvis.

Pelvic Floor Exercises

The pelvic floor muscles play a crucial role in supporting the uterus, bladder, and bowel during pregnancy and childbirth. Strengthening these muscles can help prevent urinary incontinence, support the growing uterus, and facilitate childbirth. Here are some exercises to strengthen the pelvic floor during pregnancy:

- Kegel Exercises: Kegel exercises involve contracting and relaxing the muscles of the pelvic floor. To perform a Kegel exercise, squeeze the muscles as if you're trying to stop the flow of urine, hold for a few seconds, then release. Aim to complete 10-15 repetitions, several times per day.
- Squatting: Squatting engages the muscles of the pelvic floor and can help strengthen and tone these muscles. Stand with your feet hip-width apart and lower your body into a squat position, keeping your knees aligned over your ankles.

Hold the squat for a few seconds, then return to standing. Repeat several times, focusing on engaging the muscles of the pelvic floor.

- Pelvic Floor Bridge: Lie on your back with your knees bent and your feet flat on the floor hip-width apart. Engage your pelvic floor muscles and lift your hips toward the ceiling, keeping your back and pelvis aligned. Hold the bridge position for a few seconds, then lower your hips back to the floor. Repeat several times to strengthen the muscles of the pelvic floor and lower back.

Exercises for Improving Posture and Reducing Swelling

Poor posture and swelling are common discomforts experienced during pregnancy, particularly in the later stages. Exercise can help improve posture, reduce swelling, and promote circulation throughout the body. Here are some exercises to improve posture and reduce swelling during pregnancy:

- Shoulder Rolls: Sit or stand tall with your shoulders relaxed and your spine elongated. Roll your shoulders up, back, and down in a circular motion, then reverse the movement. Repeat several times to release tension in the shoulders and upper back and improve posture.
- Ankle Circles: Sit or stand with your feet flat on the floor. Lift one foot off the floor and rotate your ankle in a circular motion, first clockwise and then counterclockwise. Repeat on the opposite side. Ankle circles help improve circulation and reduce swelling in the feet and ankles.
- Leg Elevation: Lie on your back with your legs elevated on a cushion or bolster, keeping your knees slightly bent. Relax your

arms by your sides and focus on deep, diaphragmatic breathing. Leg elevation promotes circulation and reduces swelling in the legs and feet, particularly after periods of prolonged standing or sitting.

Exercise Modifications for Each Trimester

As pregnancy progresses, the body undergoes significant changes that may impact exercise routines. It's important to make adjustments to accommodate these changes and ensure safety and comfort throughout each trimester. In this chapter, we'll explore exercise modifications tailored for each trimester, including adjustments for changing body and energy levels, safe exercises for the first trimester, and modifications for the second and third trimesters.

Adjustments for Changing Body and Energy Levels

Pregnancy brings about various physical and hormonal changes that can affect energy levels, comfort, and exercise tolerance. To accommodate these changes, consider the following adjustments:

- Listen to Your Body: Pay attention to how you're feeling during exercise and adjust your routine accordingly. If you're feeling fatigued or uncomfortable, scale back the intensity or duration of your workouts.
- Modify Intensity: As pregnancy progresses, you may need to decrease the intensity of your workouts to prevent overexertion and reduce the risk of injury. Focus on maintaining a moderate level of intensity that allows you to comfortably carry on a conversation during exercise.

- Incorporate Rest Days: Allow for adequate rest and recovery between workouts to prevent fatigue and promote overall well-being. Consider incorporating active recovery activities such as walking, swimming, or gentle yoga on rest days to maintain mobility and circulation.

Safe Exercises for the First Trimester

The first trimester is a critical period of fetal development, and it's important to prioritize safety and comfort during this time. While many women are able to continue their regular exercise routines during the first trimester, some modifications may be necessary to accommodate early pregnancy symptoms such as nausea and fatigue. Here are some safe exercises for the first trimester:

- Walking: Brisk walking is a safe and effective form of exercise during the first trimester. Aim to walk for at least 30 minutes most days of the week to maintain cardiovascular health and boost energy levels.

- Swimming: Swimming is a low-impact exercise that is gentle on the joints and provides a full-body workout. Consider incorporating swimming or water aerobics into your exercise routine to relieve joint pain and promote relaxation.
- Prenatal Yoga: Prenatal yoga classes often cater to the needs of pregnant women and provide modifications for early pregnancy symptoms such as nausea and fatigue. Gentle stretching and relaxation exercises can help alleviate stress and promote a sense of well-being during the first trimester.

Modifications for the Second and Third Trimesters

As pregnancy progresses into the second and third trimesters, the body undergoes additional changes that may necessitate further modifications to exercise routines. Here are some considerations for exercising safely during the second and third trimesters:

- Avoid High-Impact Activities: As the uterus grows larger and the center of gravity shifts, high-impact activities such as running and jumping may become uncomfortable or risky. Consider switching to lower-impact exercises such as walking, swimming, or stationary cycling to reduce stress on the joints and pelvic floor.
- Focus on Stability and Balance: Incorporate exercises that promote stability and balance, such as squats, lunges, and pelvic floor exercises. These exercises can help strengthen the core and improve posture, reducing the risk

of falls and injuries as the belly grows.

- Listen to Your Body: Pay close attention to how your body responds to exercise and make adjustments as needed. If you experience any discomfort, dizziness, or shortness of breath, stop exercising and consult with your healthcare provider.

Postpartum Exercise and Recovery

After childbirth, many women are eager to regain strength, fitness, and overall well-being through exercise. However, it's important to approach postpartum exercise with caution and care to promote recovery and prevent injury. In this chapter, we'll explore the importance of postpartum exercise, guidelines for gradually returning to exercise, and exercises to strengthen the core and pelvic floor after childbirth.

Importance of Postpartum Exercise

Postpartum exercise plays a crucial role in promoting physical and emotional recovery after childbirth. Regular physical activity can help:

- Restore Strength and Function: Pregnancy and childbirth place significant demands on the body, leading to changes in muscle tone, strength, and function. Postpartum exercise can help rebuild muscle strength, improve cardiovascular fitness, and restore mobility and flexibility.
- Promote Healing and Recovery: Exercise stimulates circulation and promotes healing by delivering oxygen and nutrients to injured tissues. Engaging in gentle, low-impact exercise can help reduce postpartum discomfort, alleviate

muscle tension, and promote overall recovery.

- Support Mental Health and Well-being: Physical activity has been shown to improve mood, reduce stress, and enhance overall well-being. For new mothers, exercise can provide a much-needed outlet for stress relief, boost self-esteem, and promote a sense of accomplishment during the challenging postpartum period.

Guidelines for Gradually Returning to Exercise

Returning to exercise after childbirth requires careful consideration and gradual progression to ensure safety and effectiveness. Here are some guidelines for gradually reintroducing exercise postpartum:

- Consult with Your Healthcare Provider: Before starting any postpartum exercise program,

consult with your healthcare
provider to ensure that you've
fully recovered from childbirth
and are cleared for physical
activity. Your healthcare provider
can provide personalized guidance
based on your individual health
status and any specific concerns or
complications related to childbirth.

- Start Slowly and Progress
  Gradually: Begin with gentle, low-
  impact exercises such as walking,
  gentle yoga, or postpartum-
  specific exercise classes designed
  for new mothers. Gradually
  increase the intensity, duration,
  and frequency of your workouts as
  your strength and stamina
  improve.
- Listen to Your Body: Pay attention
  to how your body responds to
  exercise and respect its signals. If
  you experience any pain,
  discomfort, or fatigue, scale back
  the intensity or duration of your
  workouts. It's important to

prioritize rest and recovery as
your body adjusts to the demands
of motherhood.

**Exercises to Strengthen the Core and
Pelvic Floor After Childbirth**

The core and pelvic floor muscles
undergo significant changes during
pregnancy and childbirth, making them
particularly important targets for
postpartum exercise. Strengthening these
muscles can help improve posture,
prevent pelvic floor dysfunction, and
reduce the risk of urinary incontinence.
Here are some exercises to strengthen the
core and pelvic floor after childbirth:

- Pelvic Floor Contractions (Kegels):
  Sit or lie comfortably and contract
  the muscles of your pelvic floor as
  if you're trying to stop the flow of
  urine. Hold the contraction for a
  few seconds, then release. Aim to
  complete 10-15 repetitions,
  several times per day, gradually

increasing the duration of the holds as your strength improves.

- Transverse Abdominis Activation: Lie on your back with your knees bent and your feet flat on the floor. Inhale deeply, then exhale as you gently draw your navel in toward your spine, engaging the deep abdominal muscles. Hold for a few seconds, then release. Repeat for several breaths, focusing on maintaining a neutral spine and pelvic alignment.

- Pelvic Tilts: Lie on your back with your knees bent and your feet flat on the floor hip-width apart. Inhale to prepare, then exhale as you gently tilt your pelvis upward, pressing your lower back into the floor. Hold for a few seconds, then release. Repeat for several breaths, focusing on engaging the muscles of the core and pelvis.

Real-life Stories and Testimonials

In this chapter, we'll hear personal accounts from women who stayed active during pregnancy, the challenges they faced, and how they overcame them. These inspirational stories highlight the journey of successful pregnancies and childbirths through exercise, providing encouragement and motivation for expectant mothers.

Personal Accounts from Women Who Stayed Active During Pregnancy

- **Sarah's Story**: Sarah shares her experience of staying active throughout her pregnancy despite experiencing fatigue and morning sickness during the first trimester. She discusses how prenatal yoga and swimming helped alleviate discomfort and maintain fitness levels throughout her pregnancy journey.

Sarah's Story: "Throughout my pregnancy, I encountered various challenges, from morning sickness to fatigue. However, I was determined to stay active for the health of both myself and my baby. Despite feeling nauseous and tired during the first trimester, I discovered that gentle exercises like walking and prenatal yoga helped alleviate my symptoms and boost my energy levels. As my pregnancy progressed, I continued to prioritize staying active, incorporating swimming and light strength training into my routine. These activities not only helped me maintain my fitness but also provided a sense of calm and relaxation amidst the changes my body was undergoing. By staying active, I felt more confident and prepared for the journey of childbirth and motherhood."

- **Emily's Journey**: Emily recounts her decision to continue running during pregnancy and the challenges she faced balancing exercise with her growing belly and changing energy levels. Despite encountering doubts and concerns from others, Emily remained committed to her fitness routine and ultimately found strength and confidence in her body's abilities.

Emily's Journey: "Running has always been my passion, so when I found out I was pregnant, I was determined to continue running for as long as I could. However, as my belly grew and my energy levels fluctuated, I faced challenges adapting my exercise routine to accommodate these changes. Despite encountering doubts and concerns from others about the safety of running during pregnancy, I listened to my body and modified my approach accordingly. Investing in supportive maternity activewear and adjusting my running technique helped reduce discomfort and maintain my confidence on the road. Ultimately, continuing to run throughout my pregnancy not only kept me physically fit but also empowered me mentally, reminding me of the strength and resilience of the female body."

- **Rachel's Experience**: Rachel shares her journey of practicing prenatal Pilates and strength training exercises to support her physical and mental well-being during pregnancy. She discusses the importance of listening to her body's cues, modifying exercises as needed, and finding a supportive community of fellow pregnant women to share experiences and encouragement.

Rachel's Experience: "During my pregnancy, I turned to prenatal Pilates and strength training to support my physical and mental well-being. As a busy working mom-to-be, finding time for exercise amidst my other responsibilities was challenging, but I knew it was essential for my health and the health of my baby. I discovered a supportive community of fellow pregnant women in my prenatal exercise classes, which provided encouragement and camaraderie throughout my journey. By listening to my body's cues and modifying exercises as needed, I was able to stay active and maintain my strength and flexibility throughout my pregnancy. Looking back, I'm grateful for the role that exercise played in preparing me for childbirth and motherhood,

instilling in me a sense of
confidence and empowerment that
carried me through labor and
delivery."

Challenges Faced and How They Overcame Them

- **Overcoming Fatigue and Nausea**:
  Many women experience fatigue
  and nausea during the first
  trimester, making it challenging to
  stay active. Through trial and
  error, Sarah discovered that gentle
  exercises such as walking and
  prenatal yoga helped alleviate
  symptoms and boost energy levels,
  allowing her to maintain her
  exercise routine.
  "The first trimester of pregnancy
  brought with it intense fatigue and
  nausea, making it difficult to stay
  active. However, I refused to let
  these symptoms derail my exercise
  routine entirely. Instead, I

experimented with different forms of low-impact exercise like walking and gentle yoga, which helped alleviate my symptoms and boost my energy levels. By listening to my body and honoring its needs, I found ways to stay active while still giving myself the rest and care I needed during this early stage of pregnancy."

- **Adapting to Changing Body**: As the belly grows and the body changes during pregnancy, women may face challenges adapting their exercise routines to accommodate these changes. Emily found creative solutions such as investing in supportive maternity activewear and modifying her running technique to reduce impact and discomfort as her pregnancy progressed.
"As my pregnancy progressed, I encountered new challenges related to my changing body.

Running, once a source of joy and freedom, became increasingly uncomfortable as my belly grew larger. However, rather than giving up on exercise altogether, I sought out alternative forms of physical activity that better suited my evolving needs. Embracing activities like swimming and prenatal Pilates allowed me to maintain my fitness and connection to my body throughout my pregnancy, reminding me that staying active is about more than just reaching a finish line—it's about nurturing and honoring the incredible journey of pregnancy."

- **Managing Time and Priorities**: Balancing exercise with work, family responsibilities, and other commitments can be challenging for pregnant women. Rachel found success by prioritizing self-care and carving out dedicated time for exercise, whether it be early morning walks, lunchtime Pilates classes, or evening stretching sessions.

"Balancing exercise with the demands of work, family, and other responsibilities was perhaps one of the greatest challenges I faced during pregnancy. However, I quickly realized that making time for self-care and exercise wasn't just a luxury—it was a necessity. By prioritizing my well-being and carving out dedicated time for exercise, I discovered a newfound sense of strength and resilience that carried me through the ups and downs of pregnancy and childbirth. From early morning walks to lunchtime yoga classes, these moments of movement and mindfulness became anchors of stability and serenity amidst the whirlwind of new motherhood."

Inspirational Stories of Successful

Pregnancies and Childbirths Through Exercise

- **Celebrating Birth Achievements**: Sarah shares the joy of completing a prenatal yoga class just days before giving birth and the sense of accomplishment she felt in staying active throughout her pregnancy. She credits regular exercise with helping her prepare mentally and physically for childbirth and motherhood. "As I reflect on my pregnancy journey, I'm filled with gratitude for the strength and resilience I discovered through exercise. Completing a prenatal yoga class just days before giving birth was a powerful reminder of the incredible capabilities of the female body. In those moments of movement and meditation, I felt connected to myself and my baby in a profound way, preparing me mentally and physically for the challenges and joys of childbirth. Giving birth was one of the most transformative experiences of my life, and I'm grateful for the role that exercise played in helping me navigate this journey with grace and confidence."

- **Empowering Birth Experiences**: Emily recounts the empowering experience of giving birth naturally after staying active and fit throughout her pregnancy. She credits her endurance and strength gained from running and strength training with helping her navigate labor and delivery with confidence and determination. "Giving birth naturally after staying active throughout my pregnancy was an empowering experience that I'll never forget. As I labored, I drew upon the endurance and strength I had gained from months of running and strength training, channeling that energy into each contraction. Despite the intensity of labor, I felt a deep sense of trust in my body's ability to birth my baby—a trust that was cultivated and strengthened through countless miles on the road and hours in the gym. In the end, I emerged from childbirth feeling empowered and exhilarated, grateful for the physical and mental resilience that exercise had instilled in me."

- **Finding Strength and Resilience**: Rachel reflects on the resilience and strength she discovered through her prenatal exercise journey and the profound impact it had on her pregnancy and childbirth experience. Despite facing challenges and uncertainties along the way, Rachel emerged from childbirth feeling empowered, confident, and ready to embrace motherhood. "Throughout my pregnancy, exercise became a source of strength and resilience that carried me through the challenges of pregnancy and childbirth. From prenatal Pilates classes to solo walks in nature, each moment of movement reminded me of the incredible capabilities of my body and the profound connection I shared with my baby. As I navigated the ups and downs of pregnancy and labor, I drew upon the physical and mental fortitude I had cultivated through exercise, emerging from childbirth feeling empowered, confident, and deeply grateful for the journey that had brought me to this moment."

As we conclude this book, let us reflect on the journey we've embarked upon together—a journey filled with invaluable insights, practical guidance, and inspiring stories of strength and resilience. From exploring the benefits of exercise during pregnancy to navigating the challenges and triumphs of postpartum recovery, we've delved into the multifaceted world of maternal health and wellness with care and compassion.

As you close these pages, may you carry with you a newfound sense of empowerment and confidence in your ability to nurture both your own well-being and that of your growing family. Remember, whether you're embarking on the adventure of pregnancy, navigating the joys and challenges of motherhood, or simply seeking to prioritize your health and happiness, you are not alone.

Let this book serve as a guiding light on your journey—a source of wisdom, encouragement, and inspiration to fuel your path forward. May you embrace each moment with courage, grace, and an unwavering belief in the incredible strength of the human spirit.

As you continue on your unique and
beautiful journey, may you find joy in the
journey, strength in the challenges, and
peace in the moments of quiet reflection.
And may the lessons learned within these
pages stay with you always, guiding you
toward a future filled with health,
happiness, and boundless possibility.

With warmest wishes for a journey filled
with love, laughter, and abundant
blessings,

9 798326 661562